CIRCLE OF SUPPORT

~Veronica Mason DNP-FNP-BC~

Quanaah Publishing

www.quanaah-publishing.com

Circle of Support

©Copyright 2014
Quanaah Publishing

Written by Dr. Veronica Mason
Edited by Steven Napoli and S. Quanaah
Cover Design by S. Quanaah

-FOR TRAINING AND PUBLIC SPEAKING INFO-

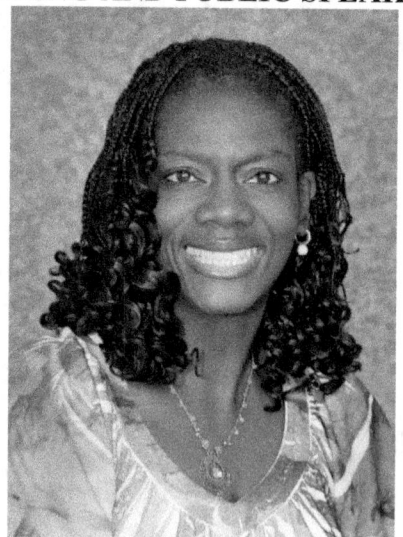

Dr. Veronica Mason
EMAIL: masonfamilymedicine@roadrunner.com

Printed in
The United States of America

Acknowledgment

A Special Thank You to Dr. Lisa Ball who prompted the initial writing of this manuscript

Introduction

The purpose of this book is to share a practice-based theoretical framework related to the use of traditional and non-traditional therapies to treat patients with chronic pain. The theoretical framework was developed within the context of a personal philosophy of nursing and other established theories, and professional practice experience to help guide provider care decisions.

-Dr. Veronica Mason

Worldview

The patient should be viewed as a whole not parts of a whole; health and wholeness are more than just absences of disease. They are a dynamic equilibrium of all the elements of one's life: healthy relationships, a fulfilling career, regular exercise, and a spiritual practice. All of these forces make up health.

Basic Assumptions

Each person in chronic pain will maintain and achieve the highest possible level of well-being and functioning. This will be achieved by treating the entire persons utilizing a comprehensive evaluation of pain and its causes. This is accomplished not only through considering an analgesic trial for pain control but implementing a team approach to pain treatment, which will include alternate and complementary therapies.

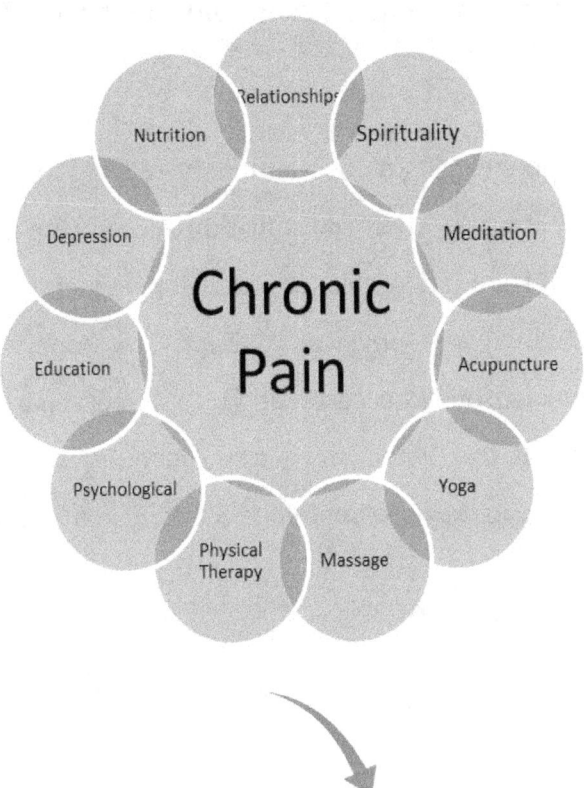

Outcome

Decreased pain, increased functional status,

and an overall increase in psychological health.

Broken Circular Line

The broken circle represents the penetrating of the protective line of defense, which can cause pain. The above areas must be addressed to bring the body back into balance.

(Adapted from Betty Neuman Systems Theory)

Step Approach Treatment to Chronic Pain

These concepts are a continuum relaxation, psychosocial, spiritual care, education and nutrition should be addresses by all and should be addresses together to achieve optimal pain control. However, physical therapy, massage, acupuncture, yoga, and chiropractic care can be utilized separately. Taking into account that when any part is incomplete or broken, the entire circle loses its completeness because all parts create the whole.

Major Concepts

Depression/Psychological

Depression can threaten the health of the entire person and must be dealt with to prevent diffuse pain. In addition, the mind can harbor bad thoughts and feelings which must be addressed and treated medically or with alternative treatment for successful reduction in pain.

Meditation

Meditation is more than the practice or relaxing, appropriate relaxation techniques can relieve feelings of anxiety or depression and create a sense of psychological wellbeing.

Nutrition

We are holistic beings as such nutrition plays an active role in each of our four parts. Advanced nutrition will foster weight loss, which will decrease pressure on the weight bearing joints causing a decrease in overall pain. In addition, adequate nutrition lifts our spirit and mental outlook.

Spiritual

Individuals who have a spiritual foundation tend to live and cope with illnesses better. Individuals who received prayer and have a spiritual foundation require fewer potent pain medications.

Acupuncture

Acupuncture is a safe, effective, natural and drug-free way to eliminate pain. Acupuncture deals with the body's vital energy circulating within the body. This promotes natural healing.

Massage Therapy

Massage therapy is an ancient therapy used to mobilize soft tissue. Massage therapy is thought to elicit a number of beneficial physiological effects, which might modulate pain; it can also relax the body, aid in tissue repair, improve blood flow in superficial vessels, elevate mood and decrease pain. Pain reduction occurs through activation of inhibitory pain pathways and by the production of endorphins.

Physical Therapy

Physical therapy has been demonstrated to be valuable techniques in pain management. It can lead to significant pain benefits, including reducing anxiety.

Education

Educating patients and family members regarding their chronic pain helps the patient take an active role in their healthcare and take ownership of their chronic pain. This will help decrease any unrealistic expectations.

Yoga

Yoga and stretching interventions that emphasize the safe performance of individual poses and special breathing techniques can minimize the risk and discomfort in patients experiencing pain.

Relationship

Having strong, supportive relationships is good for your mental and physical health.

Who is a candidate for Narcotics?

Unfortunately with the growing epidemic of opiate abuse and diversion and the tighter control of the federal government all patients must be assessed to determine if they are candidates for opiates.

Patients with recent or active addiction with current illicit substances would be better served seeking help for their addiction first with either outpatient or in patient detox prior to seeking help for pain these patients are not candidates for opiate therapy.

Patients with severe psychiatric instability must be undergoing concurrent treatment with a psychiatrist and counselor to be a candidate for opiate therapy. Research has shown that having a mental illness can make a person more likely to abuse drugs, to make their symptoms feel better in the short-term. Below is a short guideline for assessing and determining and documenting patients on opiates.

Guidelines for Assessment and Documentation

Alternative strategies for managing pain must be explored. If alternative strategies for managing the pain are unsuccessful, long-term opioid therapy can be added. The goal is not merely to treat the symptoms of pain but to devise pain management strategies that deal effectively with all aspects of the patient's pain syndrome, including psychological, physical, social, and work-related factors. Documentation in the patient's medical record should include:

History and medical examination

A complete comprehensive assessment and physical examination and comprehensive medical history must be part of the overall treatment; this includes face to face talking and observing the patient. In addition past pain treatment outcomes and any history of addiction risks to establish a diagnosis and treatment plan must be reviewed. The complete assessment should include all self-reports, review of trial of analgesics and alternative therapies, and all potential causes of pain.

Diagnosis and medical indication

A working diagnosis must be delineated, which includes the presence of a recognized medical indication for the use of any treatment or medication.

Written treatment plan with recorded measurable objectives

The plan should have clearly stated, measurable objectives, indication of further planned diagnostic evaluation, and alternative treatments. The plan should include etiology, type and severity of pain, needs, risk and goals. The provider should address underlying causes when possible, a step-wise approach to pain should be utilized which includes pharmacological and non-pharmacological interventions. The provider should document symptoms and degree of relief, monitor for effectiveness and adverse consequences and side effects.

Informed consent

Informed consent should be obtained for any injections such as trigger injections or epidurals the patient may have to undergo. In addition discussions of risks and benefits of medications should be noted in the patient's record.

Periodic reviews and modifications indicated

The provider should continually reassess the patient's treatment plan, the patient's clinical course, and outcome goals with particular attention paid to disease progression, side effects, and emergence of new conditions. Particular attention should be made not only to the patient pain but her there psychological conditions and referral a counselor or psychiatrist of warranted. In addition if evidence of aberrant medication behaviors arise this should be addressed before escalation is noted.

Records

The provider should keep accurate and complete records documenting the dates and clinical findings for all evaluations, consultations, treatments, medications, and patient instructions.

Assessment

Subjective reports by the patient should be supported by objective observations, however in there is not always a definitive cause to chronic pain. There will not always have positive MRI's or X-rays. Objective measures in the patient's condition are determined by an ongoing assessment of the patient's functional status, including the ability to engage in work or other gainful activities, patient consumption of healthcare resources, positive answers to specific questions about the pain intensity and its interference with activities of daily living, quality of family life and social activities, and physical activity of the patient as observed by the physician.

Monitoring of Patients on opioids

All patients on opioids must be monitored by providers this monitoring can take place at every visit to ensure compliance with treatment plan, to prevent diversion of medications as well as to address any unwanted side effects are occurring. Communications goes a long way and providers must explain all aspects of long-term opioid management and treatment, this includes explaining to the patient that they cannot opioids from more than one provider at a time. This should be clearly written in the pain agreement. All providers should be particularly cautious with patients who have a history of alcoholism or other drug addiction when prescribing long-term opioids. Consultation with addiction specialists is recommended.

Urine Toxicology screens

Urine toxicology screens have become an integral part of pain management practices to monitor compliance with opioid therapy and to ensure no illicit drug activity. Providers should consider testing all patients that are on opioids regardless of age this should be clearly written and explained in your pain agreement so no questions arise. A reputable urine drug screening company should be utilized one that measure quantitative levels of the medications that are detected, some companies have can detect when the patient last ingested the medication. The patients should ask when he last ingested the medication and should be documented in the patient chart. In addition it should be clearly stated and explained to the patient the consequences for have inconsistent or abnormal drug screen.

Recent I-Stop Legislation in New York State

In June of 2013 the New York state legislature passed the I-stop legislation (The Internet System for Tracking Over-Prescribing Act). The I-stop law makes New York State one of the toughest states in regards to narcotic prescribing. This legislation ushered in the PMP (prescription monitoring program) which requires all providers to access and review the patient history on the PMP before any scheduled II, III, & IV controlled substances are issued, this is considered the "Duty to Consult".

The PMP can be accessed 24 hours a day at https://commerce.health.state.ny.us and it is in "real time".

There is a Duty to consult and complying with the regulations is strictly enforced and mandatory, patients cannot op-out of the registry. Failure to comply with the PMP carries fines and penalties, including loss of license, civil penalties and/or criminal charges. The "Duty to Consult" is found at Public Health Law 3343-a, and became effective August 27, 2013. The legislation was supported by family members who have lost loved ones to prescription drug abuse. The law is intended to curtail prescription drug abuse, diversion and doctor shopping. All of this information can be found on the New York State Website (nys.gov) or the New York State DEA website.

Effective November 25, 2012 New York State changed the schedule of many controlled substances. Please see the following changes on the next page!!

Schedule II Additions:

- Tapentadol **(Nucynta)**

- Immediate precursor to fentanyl: 4-anilino-N-phenethyl-4-piperidine (ANPP)

- Hydrocodone (all products containing hydrocodone)

Schedule IV Additions:

- Carisoprodol **(Soma)**

- Tramadol **(Ultram, Ultracet, Ryzolt)**

Appendix A
(Patient Hand-Out)
Safe Protection and Storing of Opioids at Home

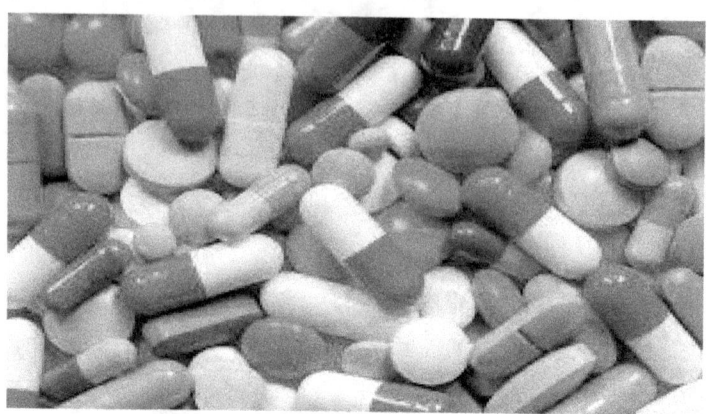

Due the increase in availability, opioid abuse has become more widespread than traditional street drugs such as cocaine, marijuana, and heroin. Many patients are unsure how to protect their medicines from theft at home here are some simple steps to take:

- Do not reveal to anyone what medications you are utilizing.
- Do not share medications with others.
- Lock all medicines especially opioids in a lock box or cabinet. These can be easily obtained for about $10 dollars at discount stores.
- Never leave medicine especially opioids in you medicine cabinet.

- Never leave medicine especially opioids on your night stand or table.
- Never leave or store opioids in your glove compartment, the heat can be unsafe.
- Never leave opioids were they are easily accessible to others such as your purse.
- Store all medicines in their original bottles with the original labels intact.
- Keep medicines out of direct sunlight to prevent the heat from degrading the medication (which can make it unsafe).
- Keep medications in a cool dry place.
- Do not crush or cut extended release medications.
- Do not cut or chew pain patches that contain opioids.
- Keep track of the medications you take to ensure you are taking them properly.

References

Astin, J. (1998). Why patients use alternative medicine. JAMA, 279(19), 1549–1553.

Bronfort, G., Haas, M., Evans, R., & Bouter, L. (2004). Efficacy of spinal manipulation and mobilization for low back and neck pain: a systemic review and best evidence synthesis. Spine, 4(3), 335-56.

Code of ethics. (2010, May 01). Retrieved from http://www.amtamassage.org/About-AMTA/Core-Documents/Code-of-ethics.html?utm_source=/about/codeofethics.html&utm_mediu m

Diego, M. A., Field, T., Hernandez-Reif, M., Hart, S., Brucker, B., & Field, T. (2001). Low back and massage therapy. International Journal of Neuroscience, 112, 122-142.

Fritz, S. (2000). Mosby's fundamentals of therapeutic massage. St. Louis, MO: Mosby.

Jagtenberg, T., Evans, S., Grant, A., Howden, I., Lewis, M., & Singer J. (2006). Evidence-based medicine and naturopathy. Journal Alternative Complement Med.12(3), 323-8.

Mao, J., Xie, S., & Bowman, M. (2010). Uncovering the expectancy effect: The validation of the acupuncture expectancy scale. Alternative Therapies, 16(6), 22-27.

Moore, R. (2009). Biobehavioral approaches to pain. Stanford, CT: Springer Publishing Company.

Paulozzi, L. U.S. Department of HHS, U.S. Department of Health and Human Services. (2008). Trends in unintentional drug overdose deaths. Retrieved from Washington, DC website http://www.hhs.gov/asl/testify/2008/03/t20080312b.html.

Pizzorno, J.E. (2005). Naturopathic medicine: A 10-year perspective (from a 35-year view). Alternative Therapy Health Med.11(2), 24-6.

Rankin-Box, D. (2002). Ethics and quality in complementary therapy education. Nursing Times, 98(2), 40-42.

Roche, G., Ponthieux, A., & Parot-Shinkel, E., (2007). Comparison of a functional restoration program with active individual physical therapy for patients with chronic low back pain: a randomized controlled trial. Physical Medicine Rehab, 88(10), 1229-35.

Sierpina, V., & Frenkel, M. (2005). Acupuncture: A clinical review. Southern Medical Journal, 98(3), 330-337.

Undefined. (2010). The White House President Barack Obama. In Office of the National Drug Control Policy. Retrieved April, 23, 2012, from http://www.whitehouse.gov/ondcp/prescription-drug-abuse.

Author Bio

Veronica Mason, DNP-MSN-FNP-BC, received her Doctorate of Nursing Practice Degree from Daemen College in Amherst NY, and her Master's Degree from D'Youville College in Buffalo, NY. Dr. Mason is a certified health coach and has been practicing in the field of pain management since 1999.

Dr. Mason, author of the '*Nurse Practitioners Guide On How To Start An Independent Practice*', is a national/international public speaker, nurse practitioner trainer, and contributing writer for local health magazines regarding the treatment of chronic pain, and various other healthcare topics. In 2009, she successfully opened, Mason Nurse Practioner in Family Medicine, PC; a pain management practice in NYS.

To Contact Dr. Mason for Interviews, Training, or Public Speaking Engagements please email her at:
masonfamilymedicine@roadrunner.com

www.ingramcontent.com/pod-product-compliance
Lightning Source LLC
Chambersburg PA
CBHW070259300526
45791CB00022B/1663